ACID REFLUX

COOKBOOK

Easy and Delicious Recipes to Prevent and Manage Acid Reflux Disease

Copyright ©2023.

This work is protected by copyright law. All rights reserved. No part of this book may be reproduced, stored in a retrieval system, transmitted in any form or by any means, electronic, mechanical, photocopying, recording, or otherwise, without the prior written consent of the copyright holder. The unauthorized reproduction, distribution, or creation of derivative works of this work is strictly prohibited and may be punishable under copyright law. The copyright holder reserves the right to pursue any and all legal remedies against any person or entity that violates the rights granted by copyright law.

TABLE OF CONTENTS

FOREWORD

My name is Sarah, and I have been living with acid reflux for as long as I can remember. I have tried various medications to help me manage my symptoms, but nothing seemed to help. That was until I decided to take matters into my own hands and look for natural solutions.

I started researching acid reflux diet recipes and lifestyle changes that might help alleviate my symptoms. After reading up on the subject, I decided to try some of the recipes that I found. I started by incorporating more fruits and vegetables into my diet, as well as cutting down on high-fat foods. I also cut back on my caffeine and alcohol consumption.

It took some time to find the right combinations of food and lifestyle changes that worked for me, but eventually, I found a combination that seemed to help. I was able to manage my acid reflux much better than before.

Inspired by my newfound success, I decided to compile all of my favorite recipes and lifestyle tips into a cookbook. I wanted to share my experiences with others who might be struggling with the same issues. I included a variety of recipes and tips on how to manage acid reflux through diet and lifestyle changes.

The cookbook was a big hit, and I have received so much positive feedback from those who have used it. It has been a great journey, and I am so glad I found something that has helped me manage my acid reflux.

I hope that my cookbook can help others who are struggling with the same issues. If you're looking for a natural way to manage your acid reflux, I highly recommend giving it a try!

Good luck!

INTRODUCTION

Are you feeling the burn of acid reflux and looking for a way to enjoy meals again? If so, you've come to the right place. This acid reflux diet cookbook is your ultimate guide to eating and cooking for acid reflux. With these delicious recipes, you'll be able to enjoy your favorite meals without the worry of heartburn. We've helped countless individuals find relief from their reflux issues by providing them with easy and tasty recipes. No matter your experience with cooking, you'll be able to create all of these dishes with ease.

In this cookbook, you will find recipes for breakfast, lunch, dinner, and snacks that are guaranteed to help you manage your acid reflux. With easy-to-follow instructions and helpful tips, you will be able to create delicious and nutritious meals that will keep you feeling your best. We've taken the guesswork out of cooking for acid reflux so you can focus on enjoying your meals. So let's get started and start reclaiming your life and your meals.

WHAT IS ACID REFLUX

Acid reflux is when the food and acid in your stomach moves back up into your esophagus. This action, which is also called acid regurgitation or gastroesophageal reflux, can cause uncomfortable symptoms like heartburn, a sour taste in the back of your throat, and chest pain.

These are other common risk factors for acid reflux disease:

- Eating large meals or lying down right after a meal
- Being overweight or obese
- Eating a heavy meal and lying on your back or bending over at the waist
- Snacking close to bedtime
- Eating certain foods, such as citrus, tomato, chocolate, mint, garlic, onions, or spicy or fatty foods
- Drinking certain beverages, such as alcohol, carbonated drinks, coffee, or tea
- Smoking
- Being pregnant

- Taking aspirin, ibuprofen, certain muscle relaxers, or blood pressure medications

What Are the Symptoms of Acid Reflux Disease?

- Heartburn: a burning pain or discomfort that may move from your stomach to your abdomen or chest, or even up into your throat
- Regurgitation: a sour or bitter-tasting acid backing up into your throat or mouth
- Other symptoms of acid reflux disease include:
- Bloating
- Bloody or black stools or bloody vomiting
- Burping
- Dysphagia -- the sensation of food being stuck in your throat
- Hiccups that don't let up
- Nausea
- Weight loss for no known reason
- Wheezing, dry cough, hoarseness, or chronic sore throat

ACID REFLUX DIET

One of the most effective ways to treat acid reflux disease is to avoid the foods and beverages that trigger symptoms. Here are other steps you can take:

- Eat smaller meals more frequently throughout the day and modify the types of foods you are eating..
- Quit smoking.
- Put blocks under the head of your bed to raise it at least 4 inches to 6 inches.
- Eat at least 2 to 3 hours before lying down.
- Try sleeping in a chair for daytime naps.
- Don't wear tight clothes or tight belts.
- If you're overweight or obese, take steps to lose
  weight with exercise and diet changes.
- Also, ask your doctor whether any medication could be triggering your heartburn or other symptoms of acid reflux disease.

ACID REFLUX DIET MEAL PLAN

DAY 1

Breakfast: Oatmeal with Bananas and Almonds

Dinner: Egg White Omelet with Spinach and Mushrooms

Lunch: Grilled Salmon with Brown Rice and Roasted Vegetables

Breakfast: Avocado Toast with Poached Egg

Lunch: Greek Yogurt Bowl with Berries and Almonds

Dinner: Grilled Chicken Breast with Quinoa and Steamed

Breakfast: Veggie Omelet with Sweet Potato Home Fries

Lunch: Roasted Turkey and Veggie Wrap

Dinner: Baked Cod with Sweet Potato Wedges and Asparagus

DAY 4

Breakfast: Low-Fat Greek Yogurt with Blueberries and Almonds

Lunch: Chickpea and Spinach Salad with Avocado

Dinner: Grilled Shrimp Skewers with Quinoa and Roasted Peppers

DAY 5

Breakfast: Oatmeal with Fresh Berries and Walnuts

Lunch: Salmon Salad with Avocado and Arugula

Dinner: Turkey Burgers with Sweet Potato Fries and Green Beans

Breakfast: Egg White Frittata with Spinach and Mushrooms

Lunch: Grilled Chicken Breast with Quinoa and Roasted Vegetables

Dinner: Vegetarian Stuffed Peppers with Brown Rice

Breakfast: Avocado Toast with Egg Whites

Lunch: Turkey and Avocado Sandwich on Whole Wheat Bread

Dinner: Baked Salmon with Brown Rice and Steamed Asparagus

ACID REFLUX RECIPES

OATMEAL WITH BANANAS AND ALMONDS

INGREDIENTS:

- 1 cup rolled oats
- 2 cups water
- 1 banana, sliced
- 1/4 cup sliced almonds
- 1 tablespoon honey (optional)

INSTRUCTIONS:

1. In a medium saucepan, bring the water to a boil.
2. Stir in the oats and reduce heat to medium-low.
3. Simmer for about 5-7 minutes, stirring occasionally, until the oats are cooked and most of the water has been absorbed.
4. Remove from heat and stir in the sliced bananas and sliced almonds.
5. Drizzle with honey if desired and serve.

GRILLED SALMON WITH BROWN RICE AND ROASTED VEGETABLES

INGREDIENTS:

- 1 pound salmon fillet
- 2 cups cooked brown rice
- 2 cups mixed vegetables (such as zucchini, bell pepper, and onion), chopped
- 1 tablespoon olive oil
- Salt and pepper, to taste

INSTRUCTIONS:

1. Preheat the grill to medium-high heat.
2. Brush the salmon fillet with olive oil and season with salt and pepper.
3. Grill the salmon for about 10-12 minutes, flipping once, until cooked through.
4. Meanwhile, toss the mixed vegetables with olive oil, salt, and pepper, and spread them on a baking sheet.
5. Roast the vegetables in a preheated oven at 400°F for about 15-20 minutes, or until tender and slightly browned.
6. Serve the grilled salmon with brown rice and roasted vegetables.

EGG WHITE OMELET WITH SPINACH AND MUSHROOMS

INGREDIENTS:

- 4 egg whites
- 1/2 cup fresh spinach, chopped
- 1/2 cup mushrooms, sliced
- 1 tablespoon olive oil
- Salt and pepper, to taste

INSTRUCTIONS:

1. In a small bowl, whisk the egg whites with salt and pepper.
2. Heat the olive oil in a nonstick skillet over medium-high heat.
3. Add the mushrooms and sauté for 2-3 minutes, until they release their moisture.
4. Add the chopped spinach and continue to sauté for another minute, until wilted.
5. Pour the egg whites over the vegetables in the skillet and let cook for 2-3 minutes, until the edges start to set.
6. Using a spatula, fold the omelet in half and continue to cook for another minute, until the egg whites are cooked through.
7. Serve hot.

AVOCADO TOAST WITH POACHED EGG

INGREDIENTS:

- 1 slice whole wheat bread, toasted
- 1/2 ripe avocado, mashed
- 1 egg
- 1 tablespoon white vinegar
- Salt and pepper, to taste

INSTRUCTIONS:

1. Fill a small saucepan with water and bring to a simmer over medium heat.
2. Add the white vinegar to the water.
3. Crack the egg into a small bowl and gently slide it into the simmering water.
4. Let the egg poach for about 3-4 minutes, until the white is set and the yolk is still runny.
5. Meanwhile, spread the mashed avocado over the toasted bread and season with salt and pepper.
6. Use a slotted spoon to remove the poached egg from the water and place it on top of the avocado toast.
7. Serve immediately.

GREEK YOGURT BOWL WITH BERRIES AND ALMONDS

INGREDIENTS:

- 1 cup plain Greek yogurt
- 1/2 cup mixed berries (such as strawberries, blueberries, and raspberries)
- 1/4 cup sliced almonds
- 1 tablespoon honey (optional)

INSTRUCTIONS:

1. In a bowl, spoon the Greek yogurt.
2. Top the yogurt with the mixed berries and sliced almonds.
3. Drizzle with honey if desired and serve.

GRILLED CHICKEN BREAST WITH QUINOA AND STEAMED VEGETABLES

INGREDIENTS:

- 1 pound boneless, skinless chicken breast
- 1 cup cooked quinoa
- 2 cups mixed vegetables (such as broccoli, carrots, and cauliflower), chopped
- 1 tablespoon olive oil
- Salt and pepper, to taste

INSTRUCTIONS:

1. Preheat the grill to medium-high heat.
2. Brush the chicken breast with olive oil and season with salt and pepper.
3. Grill the chicken for about 6-7 minutes per side, until cooked through.
4. Meanwhile, steam the mixed vegetables until tender.
5. Serve the grilled chicken with quinoa and steamed vegetables.

VEGGIE OMELET WITH SWEET POTATO HOME FRIES

INGREDIENTS:

- 2 eggs
- 1/4 cup mixed vegetables (such as bell pepper, onion, and tomato), chopped
- 1 tablespoon olive oil
- Salt and pepper, to taste
- 1 sweet potato, peeled and diced

INSTRUCTIONS:

1. In a small bowl, whisk the eggs with salt and pepper.
2. Heat the olive oil in a nonstick skillet over medium-high heat.
3. Add the chopped vegetables and sauté for 2-3 minutes, until tender.
4. Pour the beaten eggs over the vegetables in the skillet and let cook for 2-3 minutes, until the edges start to set.
5. Using a spatula, fold the omelet in half and continue to cook for another minute, until the eggs are cooked through.
6. Meanwhile, heat another tablespoon of olive oil in a separate skillet over medium-high heat.
7. Add the diced sweet potato to the skillet and season with salt and pepper.
8. Sauté the sweet potatoes for about 10-12 minutes, until tender and slightly browned.
9. Serve the veggie omelet with sweet potato home fries.

INGREDIENTS:

- 1 whole wheat wrap
- 2-3 slices roasted turkey breast
- 1/4 cup mixed vegetables (such as lettuce, tomato, and onion), chopped
- 2 tablespoons hummus
- Salt and pepper, to taste

INSTRUCTIONS:

1. Lay the whole wheat wrap on a flat surface.
2. Spread the hummus over the wrap.
3. Arrange the sliced turkey and chopped vegetables on top of the hummus.
4. Season with salt and pepper.
5. Roll the wrap tightly and serve.

BAKED COD WITH SWEET POTATO WEDGES AND ASPARAGUS

INGREDIENTS:

- 1 pound cod fillet
- 2 sweet potatoes, cut into wedges
- 1/2 pound asparagus, trimmed
- 1 tablespoon olive oil
- Salt and pepper, to taste

INSTRUCTIONS:

1. Preheat the oven to 400°F.
2. Arrange the sweet potato wedges and asparagus on a baking sheet.
3. Drizzle with olive oil and season with salt and pepper
4. Bake for 20-25 minutes, until the sweet potatoes are tender and the asparagus is crisp-tender.
5. Season the cod fillet with salt and pepper and place it on a separate baking sheet.
6. Bake the cod fillet for about 12-15 minutes, until cooked through.

7. Serve the baked cod with sweet potato wedges and asparagus.

CHICKPEA AND SPINACH SALAD WITH AVOCADO

INGREDIENTS:

- 2 cups baby spinach
- 1 can chickpeas, drained and rinsed
- 1 avocado, diced
- 1/4 cup crumbled feta cheese
- 2 tablespoons balsamic vinegar
- 1 tablespoon olive oil
- Salt and pepper, to taste

INSTRUCTIONS:

1. In a large bowl, combine the baby spinach, chickpeas, and diced avocado.
2. Add the crumbled feta cheese and toss to combine.
3. In a small bowl, whisk together the balsamic vinegar, olive oil, salt, and pepper.
4. Drizzle the dressing over the salad and toss to coat.
5. Serve the chickpea and spinach salad with avocado.

GRILLED SHRIMP SKEWERS WITH QUINOA AND ROASTED PEPPERS

INGREDIENTS:

- 1 pound large shrimp, peeled and deveined
- 1 cup cooked quinoa
- 2 roasted red peppers, sliced
- 1 tablespoon olive oil
- Salt and pepper, to taste

INSTRUCTIONS:

1. Preheat the grill to medium-high heat.
2. Thread the shrimp onto skewers and brush with olive oil.
3. Season the shrimp with salt and pepper.
4. Grill the shrimp skewers for 2-3 minutes per side, until cooked through.
5. Serve the grilled shrimp skewers with quinoa and roasted peppers.

SALMON SALAD WITH AVOCADO AND ARUGULA

INGREDIENTS:

- 1 can salmon, drained and flaked
- 1 avocado, diced
- 2 cups arugula
- 2 tablespoons lemon juice
- 1 tablespoon olive oil
- Salt and pepper, to taste

INSTRUCTIONS:

1. In a large bowl, combine the flaked salmon, diced avocado, and arugula.
2. In a small bowl, whisk together the lemon juice, olive oil, salt, and pepper.
3. Drizzle the dressing over the salmon salad and toss to coat.
4. Serve the salmon salad with avocado and arugula.

TURKEY BURGERS WITH SWEET POTATO FRIES AND GREEN BEANS

INGREDIENTS:

- 1 pound ground turkey
- 1/4 cup chopped onion
- 1/4 cup chopped fresh parsley
- 1/4 cup breadcrumbs
- 1 egg, lightly beaten
- Salt and pepper, to taste
- 2 sweet potatoes, cut into wedges
- 1 tablespoon olive oil
- 1/4 teaspoon paprika
- 1 pound green beans, trimmed
- 1 tablespoon balsamic vinegar

INSTRUCTIONS:

1. Preheat the oven to 400°F.
2. In a large bowl, combine the ground turkey, chopped onion, chopped parsley, breadcrumbs, beaten egg, salt, and pepper.
3. Mix well and shape into 4-6 patties.

4. Place the sweet potato wedges on a baking sheet, drizzle with olive oil, and sprinkle with paprika.
5. Toss to coat and bake for 20-25 minutes, until tender and crisp.
6. Meanwhile, heat a grill or grill pan to medium-high heat.
7. Grill the turkey burgers for 5-6 minutes per side, until cooked through.
8. In a large pot of boiling water, blanch the green beans for 2-3 minutes, until bright green and tender-crisp.
9. Drain and toss with balsamic vinegar.
10. Serve the turkey burgers with sweet potato fries and green beans.

EGG WHITE FRITTATA WITH SPINACH AND MUSHROOMS

INGREDIENTS:

- 8 egg whites
- 1/4 cup low-fat milk
- 1 cup fresh spinach
- 1 cup sliced mushrooms
- 1/4 cup shredded Parmesan cheese
- 1 tablespoon olive oil

- Salt and pepper, to taste

INSTRUCTIONS:

1. Preheat the broiler to high heat.
2. In a large bowl, whisk together the egg whites, low-fat milk, salt, and pepper.
3. In a large oven-safe skillet, heat the olive oil over medium-high heat.
4. Add the spinach and mushrooms and cook until tender, about 5-7 minutes.
5. Pour the egg mixture over the vegetables in the skillet.
6. Sprinkle the shredded Parmesan cheese on top.
7. Cook for 3-4 minutes, until the edges start to set.
8. Transfer the skillet to the broiler and broil for 2-3 minutes, until the top is golden and set.
9. Slice the frittata into wedges and serve.

GRILLED CHICKEN BREAST WITH QUINOA AND ROASTED VEGETABLES

INGREDIENTS:

- 4 boneless, skinless chicken breasts
- 1 cup quinoa
- 2 cups mixed vegetables (such as bell peppers, zucchini, and onion), chopped
- 2 tablespoons olive oil
- Salt and pepper, to taste

INSTRUCTIONS:

1. Preheat the grill to medium-high heat.
2. Season the chicken breasts with salt and pepper.
3. Grill the chicken breasts for 5-6 minutes per side, until cooked through.
4. Meanwhile, cook the quinoa according to package instructions.
5. In a large bowl, toss the chopped vegetables with olive oil, salt, and pepper.
6. Spread the vegetables in a single layer on a baking sheet and roast for 15-20 minutes, until tender and caramelized.

7. To serve, divide the cooked quinoa and roasted vegetables among four plates.

8. Slice the grilled chicken breasts and place on top of the quinoa and vegetables.

VEGETARIAN STUFFED PEPPERS WITH BROWN RICE

INGREDIENTS:

- 4 bell peppers, tops cut off and seeded
- 1 cup cooked brown rice
- 1 cup canned black beans, drained and rinsed
- 1/2 cup chopped onion
- 1/2 cup chopped mushrooms
- 1/2 cup chopped zucchini
- 1/2 cup chopped tomatoes
- 1/4 cup shredded cheddar cheese
- 1 tablespoon olive oil
- Salt and pepper, to taste

INSTRUCTIONS:

1. Preheat the oven to 375°F.
2. In a large bowl, combine the cooked brown rice, black beans, chopped onion, chopped mushrooms, chopped zucchini, chopped tomatoes, olive oil, salt, and pepper.
3. Mix well.
4. Stuff the mixture into the bell peppers and place the peppers in a baking dish.
5. Cover the dish with foil and bake for 40-45 minutes, until the peppers are tender.
6. Remove the foil and sprinkle the shredded cheddar cheese on top of the stuffed peppers.
7. Return the dish to the oven and bake for an additional 5-10 minutes, until the cheese is melted and bubbly.
8. Serve hot.

AVOCADO TOAST WITH EGG WHITES

INGREDIENTS:

- 2 slices whole grain bread
- 1 avocado, mashed
- 4 egg whites
- Salt and pepper, to taste

INSTRUCTIONS:

1. Toast the bread slices.
2. In a small bowl, whisk the egg whites with salt and pepper.
3. In a non-stick skillet, cook the egg whites over medium heat until set, about 3-4 minutes.
4. Spread the mashed avocado evenly over the toasted bread slices.
5. Top each slice with cooked egg whites.
6. Sprinkle with additional salt and pepper, if desired.
7. Serve immediately.

TURKEY AND AVOCADO SANDWICH ON WHOLE WHEAT BREAD

INGREDIENTS:

- 2 slices whole wheat bread
- 2 ounces sliced turkey breast
- 1/2 avocado, sliced
- 1/4 cup baby spinach leaves
- 1 tablespoon Dijon mustard

INSTRUCTIONS:

1. Toast the bread slices.
2. Spread the Dijon mustard on one slice of bread.
3. Layer the sliced turkey, avocado, and spinach leaves on top of the Dijon mustard.
4. Top with the second slice of bread.
5. Cut the sandwich in half, if desired.
6. Serve immediately.

BAKED SALMON WITH BROWN RICE AND STEAMED ASPARAGUS

INGREDIENTS:

- 4 salmon fillets
- 1 tablespoon olive oil
- 1 teaspoon garlic powder
- 1 teaspoon paprika
- 1/2 teaspoon salt
- 1/4 teaspoon black pepper
- 2 cups cooked brown rice
- 1 pound asparagus, trimmed
- 1 tablespoon butter

INSTRUCTIONS:

1. Preheat the oven to 400°F.
2. Line a baking sheet with parchment paper.
3. In a small bowl, mix together the olive oil, garlic powder, paprika, salt, and black pepper.
4. Brush the salmon fillets with the spice mixture and place them on the prepared baking sheet.

5. Bake the salmon for 12-15 minutes, until cooked through.
6. While the salmon is cooking, steam the asparagus until tender, about 5-7 minutes.
7. Toss the steamed asparagus with butter and season with salt and pepper, to taste.
8. Serve the baked salmon with brown rice and steamed asparagus.

INGREDIENTS

- 1 pear, chopped
- 2 tbsp. water
- 1/4 tsp. cinnamon (or more)
- 1/3 cup oats
- 2/3 cup unsweetened vanilla almond milk (or other milk)
- 1 tsp. maple syrup (or more)

INSTRUCTIONS

1. Stove top option: Add the pear, water, and cinnamon to a small pot.
2. Bring to a simmer and let cook for 4-6 minutes, stirring a few times, until the pears begin to become tender. (You can cook longer if you prefer the pears to break down more.) Then add the oats, milk, and maple syrup.
3. Bring back to a simmer and cook for 5-7 minutes until oats are tender. Make sure to stir a few times throughout cooking so it doesn't stick to the bottom of the pot and burn.

4. Microwave option: Add the pear, water, and cinnamon to a microwave safe bowl.

5. Microwave for 2-3 minutes until the pears are tender. (You can cook longer if you prefer the pears to break down more.) Stir in the oats, maple syrup, and milk. Microwave for 1.5 minutes.

6. Stir and microwave for another 1-1.5 minutes or until tender.

CHICKEN FRIED RICE

INGREDIENTS

- 2 tbsp.
- extra-virgin olive oil
- 3 chicken breasts (about 1 1/2 lb.)
- Kosher salt
- Freshly ground black pepper
- 2 tbsp.
- sesame oil, divided
- 1 medium onion, chopped
- 2 carrots, peeled and diced
- 3 cloves garlic, minced
- 1 tbsp freshly minced ginger
- 4 c cooked white rice (preferably leftover)

- 3/4 c frozen peas
- 3 large eggs, beaten
- 3 tbsp low-sodium soy sauce
- 2 green onions, thinly sliced

INSTRUCTIONS

1. In a medium skillet over medium heat, heat olive oil. Season chicken with salt and pepper on both sides, then add to skillet, and cook until golden and no longer pink, 8 minutes per side.
2. Remove from skillet and let rest 5 minutes, then cut into bite-sized pieces.
3. To the same skillet, heat 1 tablespoon sesame oil.
4. Add onion and carrots and cook until soft, 5 minutes, Add garlic and ginger and cook until fragrant, 1 minute more. Stir in rice and peas and cook until warmed through, 2 minutes.
5. Push rice to one side of skillet and add remaining tablespoon sesame oil to other side.
6. Add egg and stir until almost fully cooked, then fold eggs into rice.

7. Add chicken back to skillet with soy sauce
    and green onions and stir to combine.

TURKEY PINEAPPLE SPINACH MEATLOAF

INGREDIENTS

- 2 tablespoons olive oil
- 1 onion, finely chopped
- 3 #garlic cloves, minced
- 1/4 cup crushed pineapple, drained
- 10 ounces frozen chopped spinach, thawed and well well well drained
- 3/4 cup seasoned bread crumbs
- 1/2 cup parmesan cheese, grated
- 2 eggs, beaten
- 2 teaspoons dried basil
- 2 teaspoons fresh sage, minced
- 1/4 teaspoon pepper
- 1 lb ground turkey
- 1 lb Italian turkey sausage (removed from casings and crumbled)

GARNISH

- 3 pineapple rings

GLAZE (OPTIONAL) 1/4

- cup pineapple preserves
- 1 tablespoon brown sugar

INSTRUCTIONS

1. Preheat oven to 350 degrees.
2. Heat olive oil in large skillet and cook onions and garlic until tender. Remove to large bowl.
3. Add pinapples, spinach (squeezed dry), bread crumbs, cheese, eggs, basil, sage and pepper. Mix well.
4. Add turkey and turkey sausage and mix gently.
5. Form into round loaf and place in 2 quart casserole dish.
6. Bake for 40 minutes, top with pineapple rings or mix the preserves and brown sugar spread on loaf, bake 15 more minutes or until internal temperature registers 160 degrees.
7. Let stand, covered, for 15 minutes before slicing.

INGREDIENTS

- 10 oz Tail-On Shrimp (Peeled & Deveined)
- 4 oz Cremini Mushrooms
- 6 oz Carrots
- 2 cloves Garlic
- 10 oz Baby Bok Choy
- 1 Tbsp Sweet White Miso Paste
- 2 Tbsps Butter
- 1 Tbsp Rice Vinegar
- 1 Tbsp Honey
- 2 Tbsps Vegetable Demi-Glace
- ¼ tsp Crushed Red Pepper Flakes
- 1 tsp Black & White Sesame Seeds

INSTRUCTIONS

1. Prepare the ingredients & start the sauce:
2. Remove the honey from the refrigerator to bring to room temperature. Wash and dry the fresh produce.
3. Cut the mushrooms into bite-sized pieces. Peel the carrots; halve lengthwise, then thinly slice on an angle. Cut off and discard

the root ends of the bok choy; roughly chop, separating the stems and leaves. Combine the sliced carrots and chopped bok choy stems in a bowl. Peel and roughly chop 2 cloves of garlic. In a bowl, whisk together the vinegar and honey (kneading the packet before opening).

4. To make the sauce, in a separate bowl, whisk together the miso paste, demi-glace, and 2 tablespoons of water until smooth.

5. Cook the vegetables in a medium pan (nonstick, if you have one), heat 1 teaspoon of olive oil on medium-high until hot. Add the mushroom pieces in an even layer. Cook, without stirring, 2 to 3 minutes, or until lightly browned.

6. Add the prepared carrots and bok choy stems; season with salt and pepper. Cook, without stirring, 4 to 5 minutes, or until lightly browned.

7. Add the chopped garlic and as much of the red pepper flakes as you'd like, depending on how spicy you'd like the dish to be; season with salt and pepper. Cook, stirring

occasionally, 1 to 2 minutes, or until softened.

8. Add the vinegar-honey mixture. Cook, stirring occasionally, 1 to 2 minutes, or until slightly thickened. Turn off the heat; stir in the chopped bok choy leaves. Transfer to a bowl and cover with foil to keep warm. Rinse and wipe out the pan.

9. Cook the shrimp Pat the shrimp dry with paper towels; season with salt and pepper. In the same pan, heat a drizzle of olive oil on medium-high until hot. Add the seasoned shrimp. Cook, stirring occasionally, 4 to 5 minutes, or until opaque and cooked through. Leaving any browned bits (or fond) in the pan, transfer to a plate.

10. Finish the sauce & serve your dish to the pan of reserved fond, add the sauce (carefully, as the liquid may splatter).

11. Cook on medium-high, stirring constantly and scraping up any fond, 1 to 2 minutes, or until slightly thickened. Turn off the heat. Stir in the butter until melted and combined. Serve the cooked vegetables topped with

the cooked shrimp and finished sauce.
Garnish with the sesame seeds. Enjoy!

SPICY TOFU WRAPS RECIPE | VEGAN & EASY

INGREDIENTS

- 1 cup (180g) tofu, sliced thinly
- 1 onion, chopped
- 1 garlic clove, minced
- 1 tsp crushed red pepper
- 1 tsp coriander, ground
- 1 tsp cumin, ground
- 1 tsp mint, dry
- 1 tsp basil, dry
- 1 Tbsp tomato paste
- 2-3 Tbsp olive oil
- FOR THE WRAP:
- 2 tortillas
- 1 cup spinach
- 1 cup lettuce, chopped
- 1 cucumber, chopped
- 1 tomato chopped
- roasted red peppers (optional)
- a handful of olives, pitted, chopped
- 1 spicy avocado sauce

INSTRUCTIONS

1. Press the tofu, so that you get rid of as much liquid as you can.
2. Then thinly slice the tofu, add it to a large non-stick pan with 2 tbsp of olive oil and cook at medium-high heat. Stir occasionally until the tofu has a golden-brown color on each side, this took me around 7-8 minutes.
3. Add the chopped onion, minced garlic and spices. Add in one more tbsp of olive oil and stir in the tomato paste, until the tofu is covered with the spices and tomato sauce. Turn the heat off.
4. Arranging the wraps: In a tortilla start with spinach, lettuce, a few generous tbsp of the tofu you made, add some cucumber, tomatoes, olives and finish with the spicy avocado sauce.
5. Wrap it up, slice in the middle and enjoy immediately!

EGG-WHITE OMELET WITH SPINACH AND COTTAGE CHEESE

INGREDIENTS

- 3 large egg whites
- Coarse salt and ground pepper
- 1 teaspoon olive oil
- 1 cup packed baby spinach
- 1/4 cup low-fat (1%) cottage cheese
- 2 tablespoons grated Parmesan

INSTRUCTIONS

1. In a medium bowl, whisk together egg whites and 1 tablespoon water; season with salt and pepper, and set aside.
2. In a medium nonstick skillet, heat oil over medium-high.
3. Add spinach, and season with salt and pepper; cook until wilted and tender, 1 minute.
4. Add egg whites; cook until nearly set, using a flexible heatproof spatula to pull sides of omelet toward center as uncooked egg whites run underneath, 1 to 2 minutes.

5. Dollop cottage cheese on top of omelet, sprinkle with Parmesan, and season with salt and pepper.

6. Gently slide omelet onto a serving plate, folding it over on itself by tipping skillet slightly.

ALMOND BUTTER & BANANA SNACK WRAPS

INGREDIENTS

- 1 Father Sam's 80-calorie Low Carb Wheat Wrap
- 1 tablespoon creamy almond butter
- 1 small banana sliced

INSTRUCTIONS

1. Lay the wrap out flat and spread almond butter over the top.

2. Lay banana slices on the almond butter and then roll up the wrap. Enjoy.

BLUEBERRY COCONUT OVERNIGHT OATS

INGREDIENTS

- 2/3 cup rolled or quick oats
- 1 1/3 cup vanilla flavored kefir
- 1 cup fresh or frozen blueberries
- 1/2 cup flaked coconut, unsweetened
- 1/4 tsp vanilla extract
- 1/4 tsp ground cinnamon

- 1 pinch fine sea salt

INSTRUCTIONS

1. Prepare two containers with airtight lids, such as small mason jars.
2. Add all ingredients to a small mixing bowl and stir to combine.
3. Evenly divide the mixture between the two containers.
4. Seal the lid and store in the refrigerator for a minimum of 4 hours.
5. When ready to serve, top with additional ground cinnamon, coconut, or sweetener of your choice (optional).

6. Transfer to a bowl or enjoy straight from the jar.

ACID REFLUX SMOOTHIE

INGREDIENTS

- ¾ cup cashew milk
- 5 fresh basil (just leaves)
- ¼ cup fresh spinach
- ½ inch ginger root
- 1 banana (frozen)
- ½ pear
- ⅓ cup rolled oats

INSTRUCTIONS

1. Blend cashew milk, basil leaves, and spinach until smooth
2. Add remaining ingredients and blend again
3. Serve over ice for a refreshingly cool smoothie

ANTI-REFLUX ENERGIZING & HEALING MORNING SMOOTHIE

INGREDIENTS

- 1 cup coconut water
- 3/4 cup berries *or fruit of your choice
- 1 tablespoon chia seeds *optional for extra protein
- 1 tablespoon aloe vera
- 1/2 teaspoon probiotics *get the recommended dosage according to age
- 1/4 teaspoon coconut oil
- 1/4 teaspoon grated ginger

INSTRUCTIONS

1. Blend everything in a high speed blender and drink right away.

REFLUX FRIENDLY BANANA BREAD

INGREDIENTS

1. Blend together flour, baking powder, baking soda, cinnamon, and salt in a medium mixing bowl. Blend together beaten egg

whites, banana, sugar, and oil in a large
mixing bowl.

2. Stir in flour mixture into the banana mixture,
   blending only until flour mixture is
   moistened.
3. Spray an 8x4x2-inch loaf pan with nonstick
   cooking spray. Spread batter in prepared
   pan.
4. Bake in a 350 degree F oven for 45 to 50
   minutes or until a toothpick inserted near the
   center comes out clean.
5. Cool bread in the pan for approximately 10
   minutes, then remove bread from pan and
   cool it thoroughly on a wire rack.

HEARTBURN-FRIENDLY CHICKEN NOODLE SOUP RECIPE

INGREDIENTS

- 1/2 tablespoon olive oil
- 1 cup celery, trimmed and chopped (about 2
  stalks)
- 8 cups water
- 2 cups carrots, peeled and chopped (about 6
  medium carrots)
- 4 low-sodium chicken bouillon cubes

- 1/2 teaspoon thyme
- 1/2 teaspoon salt
- 3 ounces dry large egg noodles
- 2 cups boneless and skinless chicken breasts, cooked and diced
- 2 cups frozen peas

INSTRUCTIONS

1. Heat olive oil over medium-high heat in a large pot. Add chopped celery and cook until translucent.
2. Add water, carrots, chicken bouillon cubes, thyme, and salt to the pot. Bring to a boil.
3. Once boiling, add egg noodles to the pot and stir.
4. Reduce the heat to low and simmer. Cook for 8 minutes or until the noodles are tender.
5. Add the diced cooked chicken breast and frozen peas. Return to a boil.
6. Once boiling again, reduce the heat to medium-low. Cover and simmer for 5 to 10 minutes, or until the peas are warm and the soup has a flavorful aroma.
7. Serve the soup in individual bowls.

INGREDIENTS

- 1 small bag of mini potatoes
- 4 tbsp olive oil
- 1 tsp salt
- 1 tsp black pepper

INSTRUCTIONS

1. Scrub potatoes and boil them until they're soft. How long will depend on their size, so check them by feeling how easily they're penetrated with a fork or knife.
2. Drain the water and toss the potatoes with olive oil. Sprinkle with salt & pepper.
3. Place in a roasting dish at 425F for about 15 minutes.
4. Serve & enjoy!

BEST SMOOTHIE FOR ACID REFLUX

INGREDIENTS

- 1 cup unsweetened almond milk
- 1 cup pineapple chunks, frozen
- ½ cup strawberries, frozen
- 1 banana
- 1 cup spinach
- 1 tsp flaxseeds

INSTRUCTIONS

1. Simply add all ingredients to your blender jar. Blend on the highest setting until creamy and smooth. Enjoy!

ACID REFLUX-FRIENDLY SMOOTHIE

INGREDIENTS

- 1 cup kale, cut into chunks
- 1 cup mango chunks, frozen
- 1 banana
- 1 cup cantaloupe melon, cut into chunks
- ½-inch fresh ginger, peeled
- 1 ½ cup unsweetened almond milk

1. Cut the kale leaves into small chunks. Peel the ginger, if it's not organic. Place everything into your blender jar and blend until smooth. Add some ice cubes to make this smooth more refreshing. Enjoy!

ANTI-ACID REFLUX SMOOTHIE

INGREDIENTS

- 1 small beet, peeled and cut into chunks
- 1 red apple, cored and cut into chunks
- 1 stalk of celery, cut into chunks
- 1 cup carrot juice
- 1 cup unsweetened almond milk
- ½-inch fresh ginger, peeled

INSTRUCTIONS

1. After you've prepared everything, place it into your blender and blend until smooth.
2. As we're using hard and fibrous vegetables such as carrots and beets, you'll need a more high-powered blender for this smoothie.
3. For great blenders that won't break your bank account.

BANANA SMOOTHIE FOR ACID REFLUX

INGREDIENTS

- 1 ½ cups unsweetened almond milk
- 2 bananas
- 2-3 almonds
- ½ cup rolled oats
- ½ tsp vanilla extract
- a hint of cinnamon

INSTRUCTIONS

1. Place the oats at the bottom of your blender.
2. Pulse a few times until ground. Add the almond milk, bananas, vanilla extract, and cinnamon.
3. Blend until creamy and smooth. Enjoy!

SIMPLE ACID REFLUX GREEN SMOOTHIE

INGREDIENTS

- 1 cup spinach
- 1 cup of water
- ½ cup mango chunks, frozen
- 1 cup pineapple chunks, frozen
- 1 banana

INSTRUCTIONS

1. Simply place all ingredients into your blender and blend on the highest setting until smooth.
2. Add ice cubes for a more refreshing taste.

ALKALINE SMOOTHIE FOR ACID REFLUX

INGREDIENTS

- 1 ½ cup unsweetened almond milk
- ½ small beet
- 1 cup cherries, frozen or fresh
- 1 banana
- ½ cup spinach (optional)

INSTRUCTIONS

1. Prepare the beets, place everything in your blender and blitz away!

ACID REFLUX SMOOTHIE WITH PINEAPPLE

INGREDIENTS

- 1 ½ cup unsweetened almond milk
- 1 banana
- 1 cup mango chunks, frozen

- 1 cup pineapple chunks, frozen
- 1 tbsp chia seeds

INSTRUCTIONS

1. Simply place everything into your blender jar, turn your blender on.
2. Blend until smooth and creamy. Enjoy!

CREAMY PUMPKIN SOUP (ACID-REFLUX FRIENDLY)

INGREDIENTS

- 4 cups squash/pumpkin cut into cubes
- 4 cloves garlic, minced
- 1 tbsp olive oil
- 3 cups chicken broth or 1 chicken cubes and 3 cups water
- 1 cup creamy soy milk, I used Vitasoy Plus Milky
- salt and pepper to taste

INSTRUCTIONS

1. Heat olive oil in a pot, sauté the garlic until fragrant. Add the squash.
2. Pour in the chicken stock or water. Bring into a boil.

3. Puree with an immersion blender or if you
    don't have an immersion blender, let it cool
    down slightly and use a regular blender.
    Transfer back into the pot and bring to a
    boil.
4. Simmer for 5-10 minutes until thickened. If
    the soup is too thick, add more chicken stock
    as needed until desired consistency is
    reached.
5. Season with salt and pepper to taste.
6. Turn off heat and add soy milk into the
    soup. Stir.
7. Enjoy with a toast or crackers for dipping

TOASTED OATMEAL

INGREDIENTS

- 1 cup quick cook oatmeal, whole flake is
  also great, just double the cooking time
- 1/2 cup water
- 1/2 cup milk
- pinch of salt

INSTRUCTIONS

1. Add oatmeal to a saucepan. Over medium-high heat, stir it constantly for 2-3 minutes until toasted and a popcorn smell starts to appear. Don't over cook, and don't stop stirring or it will burn.
2. Add all other ingredients. Bring to boil. Lower temperature and simmer for 3-4 minutes until thickened, stirring occasionally.
3. Serve with your favourite toppings. I love yogurt, blueberries and pumpkin seeds.

FLANK STEAK WITH CHIMICHURRI

INGREDIENTS

- 1 teaspoon dried oregano
- 1 teaspoon ground cumin
- ½ teaspoon sea salt, divided
- 1 (12-ounce) flank steak
- 3 tablespoons olive oil, divided
- ½ cup chopped fresh parsley
- ¼ cup chopped fresh cilantro
- Grated zest of ½ lime

INSTRUCTIONS

1. In a small bowl, stir together the oregano, cumin, and 1⁄4 teaspoon of salt. Sprinkle evenly all over the flank steak.
2. Heat 1 tablespoon of oil in a large nonstick skillet over medium-high heat until it shimmers.
3. Add the flank steak and cook for 2 to 3 minutes per side.
4. Reduce the heat to low. Continue cooking until the steak it reaches 135°F for medium-rare, about 5 minutes more.
5. Meanwhile, in a blender or food processor, combine the remaining 2 tablespoons of oil, parsley, cilantro, lime zest, and remaining 1⁄4 teaspoon of sea salt. Pulse 20 times, or until it is well combined.
6. Slice the flank steak thinly slices against the grain. Serve with the chimichurri.

INGREDIENTS

- 3 units chicken breasts
- 1 units chicken broth
- 612 tablespoons green onions
- 1 units butter or margarine
- 3 ounces cream cheese
- 1 cups milk
- 8 ounces sour cream
- 0.25 teaspoons ground comino
- 10 ounces mushroom soup
- 1020 units tortillas
- 1 units shredded cheese
- 1 units pepper
- 1 units garlic powder
- 1 units onion powder
- 1 units ground pepper
- 1 units salt
- 1 units comino

INSTRUCTIONS

1. Boil chicken until fully cooked. You can add any seasonings you want to the water/broth,

to give it more flavor. I use pepper, garlic powder, ground comino and onion powder. Once cooked, drain water/broth, let chicken cool and shred into bite size pieces.

2. In a pan, cook chopped green onions in butter. Cook just until they start to wilt. Drain remaining butter or margarine. In bowl mix cream cheese, chicken, 1 Tbsp. milk, sour cream, comino, and green onions. In a separate bowl mix the cream of mushroom soup with 1 cup of milk.

3. Line your pan with foil. In each tortilla fill with the cream cheese, chicken mixture from bowl 1. Be sure not to over fill the tortilla so it will roll closed. After each is closed, put in pan. When all tortillas are filled and are in the pan, pour cream of mushroom soup from bowl 2 over all tortillas in the pan. Cover with foil.

4. Put in the oven at 350°F for 35 minutes. Take out and add shredded cheese. Put back into the oven for 5-7 minutes. Enjoy!!

INGREDIENTS

- 1 28-Ounce Can San Marzano Tomatoes - Crushed
- 1/2 Cup Mineral Water -Mineral Water is highly alkaline
- 3 Cloves Garlic -Optional, crushed and chopped
- 3 Tablespoons Olive Oil
- 3/4 Cup Carrots -Finely grated
- 1/4 Cup Celery -Finely grated
- 8 Ounces Mushrooms -Optional, finely chopped
- 1 Teaspoon Baking Soda
  - 1/2 Teaspoons Salt
- 1/2 Teaspoon Red Pepper Flakes
- Teaspoons Dried Oregano
- Teaspoons Dried Basil -or 1/4 cup fresh basil, roughly chopped
- 1 Tablespoon Tomato Paste

INSTRUCTIONS

1. In a large bowl, carefully crush the tomatoes by hand, they will squirt everywhere, so be gentle or you'll be covered in tomato juice
2. Rinse can with water to get all the sauce
3. In a large skillet, heat the olive oil over medium-high heat, add the garlic and the tomato paste and cook briefly, just to get the raw flavor out of it, approximately 30-45 seconds
4. Add the crushed tomatoes and sauce, and all remaining ingredients, unless you're using fresh basil, then add it at the end after the heat is off
5. Bring to a simmer, stirring frequently, simmer for approximately 30 minutes

ACID-REFLUX FRIENDLY FISH

INGREDIENTS

- cod fish fillets
- 1/2 cup 1% low-fat milk
- seasoning
- sheets kitchen aluminum foil
- 1 tablespoon dried herbs

INSTRUCTIONS

1 Preheat oven.

2 Lay the cod fillets on the foil sheets.

3 Season lightly, and sprinkle on the herbs.

4 Bend up the sides of the foil to make 'nests' but don't close yet.

5 Pour half the milk into each nest.

6 Seal the foil packages.

7 Bake for 20mins or according to instructions on fish.

8 Serve with potatoes mashed with milk and a little low-fat spread, plus whatever vegetable the sufferer can tolerate. NB - if only one person in your family has acid reflux, you can put whatever flavouring you like in the other packages, such as ginger, garlic or curry powder.

INGREDIENTS

- 2 Tbsp extra-virgin olive oil, plus more for garnish
- 1 small fennel bulb thinly sliced (save fronds for garnish)
- Salt and freshly ground black pepper, to taste
- 1 small bunch Swiss chard, stemmed, cleaned and torn into bite-size pieces
- flour, for dusting
- 8 oz refrigerated pizza dough, at room temperature
- cornmeal, for dusting
- 1/3 cup cauliflower Alfredo sauce (such as Ragu)
- 1/2 cup shredded smoked Gouda or provolone cheese
- 1/2 cup shredded cooked chicken breast
- grated Parmigiano-Reggiano cheese, for garnish (optional)
- flake sea salt, for garnish (optional)

INSTRUCTIONS

1   One hour before baking, place a pizza stone on rack in top third of oven. Preheat oven to 500°F.

2   In a large skillet, heat oil over medium-high. Add fennel, salt and pepper. Saute 3–4 minutes or until tender.

3   Stir in chard. Saute 2–3 minutes or until chard is wilted and tender. Set aside.

4   On a lightly floured work surface, use your hands or a rolling pin to shape dough into a 12-inch circle.

5   Transfer dough to a pizza peel or rimless cookie sheet dusted with cornmeal. Spread with sauce. Top with smoked Gouda, chard mixture and chicken. Bake 8–10 minutes or until cheese is bubbly and crust is browned. Drizzle with additional olive oil.

6   If desired, sprinkle with Parmigiano-Reggiano, flake sea salt and fennel fronds.

INGREDIENTS

- 172 g quinoa (uncooked, rinsed thoroughly. Seriously, rinse it really good, otherwise it will end up tasting bitter) - for IBS, avoid whole grain. Use white quinoa instead
- 1+1/2 cups water
- 1/2 tsp. salt (I use Pink Rose Himalayan Salt)
- 1 Tbsp. garlic-infused olive oil (see notes section regarding this product)
- 1/4 cup+1 Tbsp. fresh chives (chopped)
- 60 g baby spinach (raw) - 60g = ~4 unpacked cups or ~2 packed cups
- 2 oz crumbled feta cheese (try and find one that is relatively low fat. The one I used and that was used for calculating nutritional information below is this one)

INSTRUCTIONS

1 Place the quinoa, water and salt in a medium-sized saucepan and heat over medium-high heat until it just begins to boil.

2   When it starts to boil, cover the pan, reduce
     heat to low and cook covered for 15 minutes.

3   When the quinoa has ~5 minutes left to cook,
     heat the oil in a medium-sized skillet over
     medium heat.

4   When the oil is heated, add the chives and
     spinach and cook, stirring constantly, until
     spinach wilts.

5   At this point the quinoa should be done.
     Remove the lid and fluff up the quinoa, then
     add in the spinach/chive mixture and the feta
     cheese and stir to incorporate everything and
     melt some of the cheese.

6   Serve this as a side dish to accompany your
     favorite entree or eat by itself as a meal as is
     for vegetarians or, for non-vegetarians, feel
     free to throw in a little chopped-up cooked
     boneless, skinless chicken breast (no more than
     3g for IBS).

SPAGHETTI SQUASH WITH ROASTED EGGPLANT, FRESH ZUCCHINI, CAPERS, AND ITALIAN TUNA

INGREDIENTS

- 3 tablespoons olive oil, plus more for drizzling
- 1 smallish spaghetti squash
- 1 smallish eggplant
- 2 heaping tablespoons of capers, chopped
- 1/2 zucchini, julienned
- 1 jar of italian tuna, drained of olive oil
- 2 cups mixed greens, air dried and coarsely chopped

INSTRUCTIONS

1 Preheat oven to 400 degrees. Line a rimmed baking sheet with parchment paper. Cut eggplant into good-sized chunks and toss with 2 Tbs. olive oil, salt and pepper to taste. Roast for about 30 – 40 minutes until lightly browned and fork tender.

2 At the same time, cut the spaghetti squash in half lengthwise and scrap out seeds and pulp and discard. Take 1 Tbs. of olive oil and coat the edges and inside of each squash half, spreading it around with your fingers. Put 1/4"

of water in a baking pan and place squash cut side down in the pan of water. Roast for 40 minutes in this position, then turn the squash over and roast for 10 – 15 minutes more, until squash is very tender, testing with a fork.

3   While eggplant and squash are roasting, drain and chop the capers. Drain the tuna and flake. Wash, air dry and coarsely chop the greens.

4   When squash is done, remove from the shell, using a fork to create the "spaghetti" and toss with the eggplant, the zucchini, capers, tuna and greens. Season with salt and pepper to taste. Drizzle olive oil on top and sprinkle on some drops of sherry vinegar.

REFLUX BANANA-ALOE SMOOTHIE

INGREDIENTS:

- 4oz - Aloe Vera Juice from inner fillet
- 1c - Skim Milk or Soy/Nut/Rice Milk
- - Bananas, frozen
- 1tbsp - Ginger Preserves (OR 1-3 tsp grated ginger and
- 1tbsp sweetner of choice.)
- 1tbsp - Agave nectar (or to taste)

- 1tbsp - Aloe Vera (If you can't find the plant, just substitute one more ounces of aloe juice.)
- 4-5 - Ice Cubes

INSTRUCTIONS

1. Put everything in a blender and blend until smooth.

COCONUT RICE

INGREDIENTS

- 2 Tbsp butter
- 1 cup sliced red onion
- 2 Tbsp chopped garlic
- 1 cup basmati rice
- 1 can, 400mL coconut milk
- 1/2 cup water
- 1/2 cup shredded toasted coconut
- 1/4 cup golden raisins
- 1/2 cup chopped fresh mint

INSTRUCTIONS

2. Heat butter in a pan over medium-high heat. Add red onion and chopped garlic, sauté 2-3 minutes. Add basmati rice, stir to coat.

3. Add coconut milk and water to the pan. Bring to boil, cover, reduce heat and simmer for 10-15 minutes until rice is tender.
4. Stir in coconut, golden raisins. Mix in (or sprinkle on top as shown) chopped fresh mint. Fluff and serve.

ACID REFLUX FRIENDLY RECIPE TUNA CASSEROLE

INGREDIENTS

- 1 (12 oz) package egg noodles
- 1 can tuna (7 oz in water)
- 1 cup frozen peas (thawed)
- 1 can (10-3/4 oz) reduced-fat cream of mushroom soup
- 1/4 cup fat-free plain yogurt
- 1/2 cup fat-free milk
- 1 TBSP Dijon mustard
- 1/4 tsp pepper
- 1/4 tsp dried basil
- 2 oz low-fat shredded cheddar
- crushed "baked" potato chips
- Fresh parsley

INSTRUCTIONS

1   Boil noodles according to package directions.
2   Drain and flake tuna.
3   In a medium bowl, mix together soup, milk, yogurt, and mustard.
4   Stir in tuna and peas.
5   Place mixture into a 9-inch round baking dish, and gently stir in noodles.
6   Mix the cheese and chips together and sprinkle over the dish.
7   Bake at 350 degrees for 30 minutes.
8   If desired, sprinkle each serving with some fresh parsley.

SIMPLE CAULIFLOWER "RICE" BRYAN

INGREDIENTS

- cups cauliflower "rice" (1/2 large head of cauliflower)
- 1 tablespoon coconut oil
- 1 cup chopped mushrooms (I used oyster but any will do)
- 1/2 teaspoon onion powder*
- 1/2 teaspoon garlic powder*
- 1 teaspoon turmeric

- 1/2 teaspoon cumin
- 1/3 cup raisins
- 2 tablespoons nutritional yeast
- 2/3 cup coconut milk (or other nut or seed milk)
- salt and pepper (to taste)

INSTRUCTIONS

1. Pulse cauliflower in a blender or food processor until it resembles rice!
2. Heat the coconut oil in a large pan over medium heat and add mushrooms and onion and garlic powders. Sauté 3-5 minutes until mushrooms start to release their water.
3. Add cauliflower rice and stir to combine with mushrooms. Add turmeric and cumin, cover and let simmer for 5-7 minutes, stirring occasionally.
4. Add raisins, nutritional yeast, and coconut milk.
5. Stir to combine and cook until the liquid has cooked out (about 5 more minutes).
6. Add salt and pepper to your taste and serve!

SIMPLE BROILED HADDOCK

INGREDIENTS

- cooking spray
- 2 pounds haddock fillets
- ½ teaspoon onion powder
- ½ teaspoon paprika
- ½ teaspoon garlic powder
- ½ teaspoon ground black pepper
- ½ teaspoon salt
- ¼ teaspoon cayenne pepper
- 1 tablespoon butter, cut in small pieces
- 1 lemon, cut into wedges

INSTRUCTIONS

1. Set oven rack about 6 inches from the heat source and preheat the oven's broiler. Line a baking sheet with aluminum foil and spray with cooking spray.
2. Arrange haddock fillets on the prepared baking sheet. Mix onion powder, paprika, garlic powder, salt, black pepper, and cayenne pepper in a small bowl; sprinkle seasoning over haddock. Dot haddock with pieces of butter.

3. Broil in the preheated oven until fish is easily flaked with a fork, 6 to 8 minutes. Serve with lemon wedges.

BUCKWHEAT AND BUTTERNUT SqUASH SALAD

INGREDIENTS

- 1 cup dry buckwheat(best soaked for 8-12h with 1 T apple vinegar, than rinsed with cold water)
- 1 small butternut squash (peeled, seeded and cut into 2 cm cubes)
- 100 g soft goat cheese
- 1 handfull of dried cherries and cranberries
- 100 g sunflower seeds

FOR THE BUTTERNUT:

- 1 T allspice
- 1 T cloves
- 1 T cardamom pods
- olive oil
- salt

VINAIGRETTE:

- 2 T apple vinegar

- 1T Dijon mustard
- 2T tahini
- 2T maple syrup

INSTRUCTIONS

1. Preheat the oven to 180C. In a spice grinder grind allspice, cloves and cardamom.
2. In a bowl toss butternut cubes with olive oil, salt and spices. Put on a baking sheet and bake for 35-40 minutes or until tender.
3. Cook buckwheat with 2 cups of water. It takes me about 15 minutes. Drain and rinse with cold water.
4. In a bowl mix buckwheat, dry cherries, butternut squash, goat cheese. In another bowl or a jar mix mustard, apple cider, maple syrup, tahini and a teaspoon of sea salt. Add to the big bowl and toss with two spoons. Sprinkle with sunflower seeds and serve.

INGREDIENTS

- piecessalmon (skinless, each about 200 grams)
- 1lemon (organic)
- salt
- freshly ground peppers
- 100 gramsbutter
- 400 gramssauerkraut (canned)
- 250 millilitersriesling
- 150 gramscrème fraiche
- 50 gramswhipped cream
- lemons (for garnishing)

INSTRUCTIONS

1. Rinse lemon in hot water, grate zest and squeeze juice.
2. Drizzle salmon with lemon juice and season with salt and pepper.
3. Heat butter in a small saucepan, season with 1/4 teaspoon of salt and allow to foam.
4. Take sauerkraut out of the can and loosen.
5. Spread about 1/3 of sauerkraut in buttered baking pan loosely, sprinkle with about 1/3

of lemon zest and top with 2 pieces of salmon. Dot fish with butter. Repeat layers, finishing with sauerkraut.

6. Whisk wine with crème fraîche and cream, season with salt and pepper and pour over gratin. Sprinkle with remaining lemon zest.

7. Bake in preheated oven at 200°C (approximately 400°F) for about 30-40 minutes. Garnish with lemon wedges and serve.

8. If desired, serve with parsley or boiled potatoes.

COCONUT TURMERIC CAULIFLOWER

INGREDIENTS

- 1 head of Cauliflower, cut into medium florets
- 1 Tbsp coconut oil (or canola or olive) oil
- 1/2 cup coconut milk (from a can)
- 1 Tbsp Piquant Post Turmeric Gold Spice blend
- salt and pepper to taste (optional)

INSTRUCTIONS

1   Preheat oven to 400. Line a sheet pan with foil. Heat a small sauté pan or skillet on Med-Low and add oil to pan. Prepare cauliflower and cut into bite-sized florets.

2   When oil heats up add Turmeric Gold spice to pan and briefly stir in the spices. Add the coconut milk and stir to mix. Bring to a low simmer for 1 minute.

3   Remove pan from heat. In a large mixing bowl add the cauliflower and pour over the coconut turmeric sauce. Using a slotted spoon, mix the cauliflower to thoroughly coat the florets.

4   Spread the cauliflower evenly on the foil and place pan in oven. Cook for 20 minutes or until soft enough to pierce with a fork.

PECAN PIE BITES

INGREDIENTS

- Cooking spray
- 1/2 c. firmly packed brown sugar
- tbsp. unsalted butter, softened
- large egg (yolk only)
- 1/2 tsp. vanillla

- 1 c. plus 2 tablespoons all-purpose flour
- 1/2 tsp. baking powder
- 1/4 tsp. salt

FOR THE FILLING:

1 c. finely chopped pecans

1/2 c. firmly packed brown sugar

1/4 c. heavy whipping cream

1 tsp. vanilla

INSTRUCTIONS

1. Preheat the oven to 350°. Spray 36 mini muffin pan cups with nonstick cooking spray; set aside.
2. Combine the brown sugar, butter, egg yolk and vanilla in a bowl. Beat with a mixer on medium speed, scraping the bowl often, until creamy. Add the flour, baking powder and salt; beat on low speed until well mixed.
3. Shape the dough into 3/4-inch balls; place each into a prepared mini muffin pan cup, pressing the dough onto bottom and up one-

third of the sides of each cup, creating a shallow cup.

4. Combine all of the filling ingredients in a bowl; spoon 1 teaspoon filling into each cookie.

5. Bake 13 to 15 minutes or until edges are golden brown. Let cool 10 minutes in the pan on a cooling rack. Remove the cookies from the pans by running a small knife around the edge of each cookie. Place onto the cooling rack; cool completely.

CONCLUSION

The GERD-Friendly Kitchen is a great resource for anyone looking to manage their acid reflux and find healthier recipes to help reduce the symptoms. With its comprehensive information and helpful tips, it is a must-have for anyone looking to improve their diet and reduce their acid reflux. With its easy to follow recipes and tips on dietary changes, this book is sure to help you make positive changes in your diet and lifestyle and lead to a healthier, happier life.

In conclusion, The GERD-Friendly Kitchen is a helpful resource for anyone looking to reduce the symptoms of acid reflux and find healthier recipes. With its comprehensive information and easy to follow recipes, it can help you make positive changes in your diet that can lead to better health and well-being.

We recommend this book for anyone who is looking for a comprehensive guide to help manage and reduce the symptoms of acid reflux.

www.ingramcontent.com/pod-product-compliance
Lightning Source LLC
Chambersburg PA
CBHW071601270726

48661CB00017B/344